7 Cloves Tips Every Woman Should Know

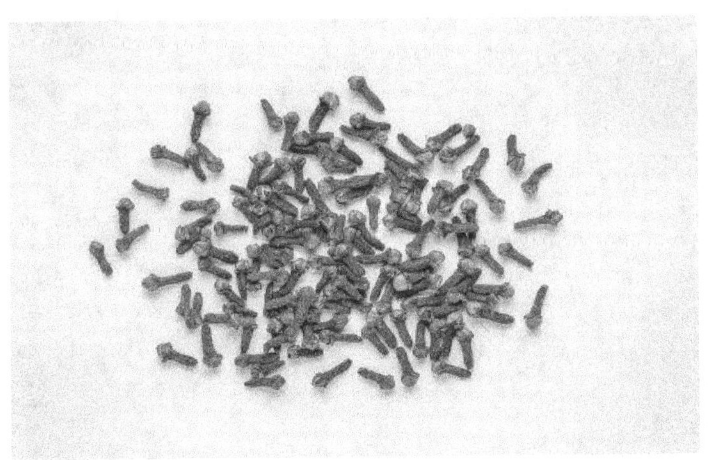

Ryan V. Lincoln

Copyright © [2023] Ryan V. Lincoln

4

<u>Table of Contents</u>

Introduction
 The Power of Cloves
How Cloves Can Improve Your
Health and Well-being

Chapter 1: Cloves for Beauty
* Cloves for Skin Health
* Cloves for Hair Health
* Cloves for Oral Health

Chapter 2: Cloves for Health
* Cloves for Immune System
Support
* Cloves for Digestive Health

* Cloves for Respiratory Health
* Cloves for Cardiovascular Health

Chapter 3: Cloves for Emotional Well-being

* Cloves for Stress Relief
* Cloves for Anxiety Relief
* Cloves for Mood Enhancement

Chapter 4: Cloves in the Kitchen

* Cooking with Cloves
* Baking with Cloves
* Making Clove-infused Beverages

Chapter 5: Cloves for Natural Remedies

* Cloves for Toothaches
* Cloves for Colds and Flu
* Cloves for Headaches
* Cloves for Stomach Upset

Chapter 6: Cloves in Aromatherapy

* Using Cloves Essential Oil for Relaxation
* Using Cloves Essential Oil for Pain Relief
* Using Cloves Essential Oil for Infection Prevention

Chapter 7: Cloves in Everyday Life

* Adding Cloves to Your Daily Routine
* Making Cloves a Part of Your Self-care Ritual
* Sharing the Benefits of Cloves with Others

Conclusion

* The Many Benefits of Cloves
* Embracing the Power of Cloves for a Healthier, Happier Life

What Is Cloves?

Cloves are the dried flower buds of a tree in the Myrtaceae family, Syzygium aromaticum. Originating from the Indonesian Maluku Islands, sometimes known as the Moluccas, they are frequently used as a spice, flavoring, or scent in commercial goods like toothpaste, soaps, and makeup. Because different countries have distinct harvest seasons, cloves are accessible all year round.

Cloves have a warm, pungent flavor and aroma that is due to

their high concentration of eugenol, an essential oil. Eugenol has a variety of medicinal properties, including anti-inflammatory, analgesic, and antiseptic properties. Cloves have been used in traditional medicine for centuries to treat a variety of ailments, including toothaches, headaches, and stomach upset.

Introduction

Embark on a journey of holistic wellness with 7 Cloves Tips Every Woman Should Know

History of Cloves

Cloves, the dried flower buds of the clove tree (Syzygium aromaticum), have a long and fascinating history, spanning centuries of trade, cultural significance, and medicinal use. Native to the Maluku Islands of Indonesia, cloves were once

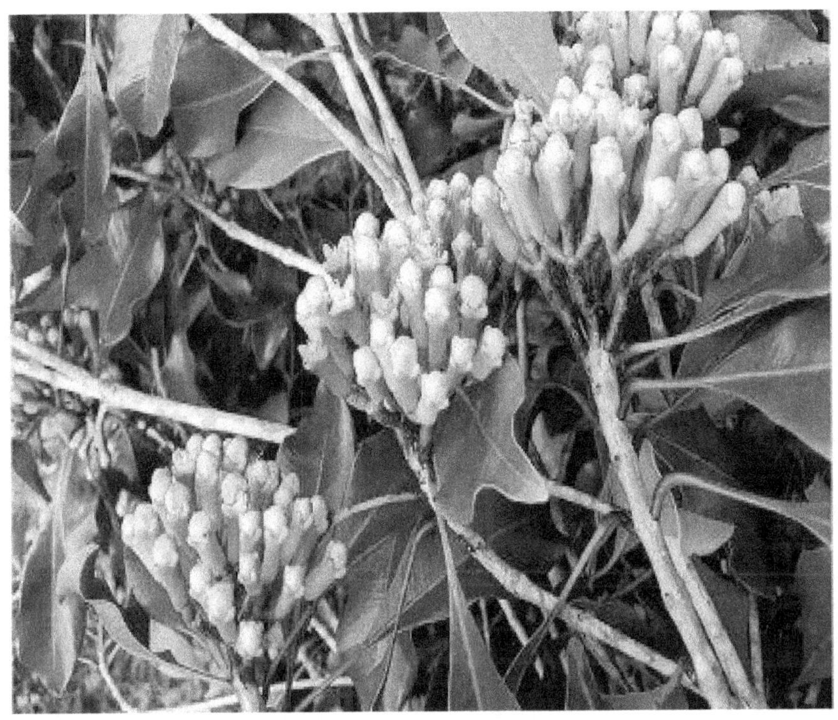

among the most valuable spices in the world, driving explorers to venture across treacherous seas in search of their exotic flavor and aroma.

<u>Early Trade and Cultural Importance</u>

The earliest records of clove trade date back to the 3rd century BC, when Chinese traders brought them from the Maluku Islands to China. From there, cloves spread along the Silk Road, reaching India, Persia, and the Mediterranean region. Their strong, pungent flavor and aroma made them highly sought after by chefs and perfumers, and their medicinal properties were also widely recognized.

European Exploration and Colonialism

In the 15th century, European explorers, driven by the lucrative spice trade, began venturing into the Indian Ocean, seeking to establish direct trade routes with clove-producing regions. The Dutch East India Company (VOC) emerged as a dominant force in the clove trade, establishing a monopoly on clove production in the Maluku Islands. This monopoly allowed the VOC to control the supply of cloves and maintain high prices, making cloves one of the most valuable commodities in Europe.

Expansion of Clove Cultivation

The high demand for cloves led to the expansion of clove cultivation beyond the Maluku Islands. In the 18th century, clove trees were successfully planted in Zanzibar, Tanzania, and other tropical regions, diversifying the supply of cloves and reducing the VOC's control over the market.

Current Production and Uses

Today, cloves are still cultivated in several tropical regions, with Indonesia, Tanzania, and Madagascar being the leading producers. Cloves remain an important spice in both culinary and medicinal applications. In cooking, cloves are used to flavor a variety of dishes, particularly meats, curries, and baked goods. Their antimicrobial properties make them a valuable ingredient in traditional medicine, and they are also used in aromatherapy and as a natural pest repellent.

Future Prospects

The global demand for cloves is expected to continue to grow, driven by increasing consumer interest in natural and traditional ingredients. The expansion of clove cultivation in new regions and the development of new applications for cloves are likely to further support the growth of the clove market.

Note that, cloves have a rich history that is intertwined with trade, exploration, and cultural significance. Their unique flavor, aroma, and medicinal properties have made them a valuable commodity for centuries, and their continued demand is likely to ensure their place in the global spice market for years to come.

In the realm of natural remedies, few herbs possess the profound potency of cloves. These aromatic buds, harvested from the Syzygium aromaticum tree, hold within them an extraordinary treasure trove of health-enhancing properties. From ancient times, cloves have been revered for their ability to promote well-being and vitality in women of all ages.

<u>Unveiling the Power of Cloves</u>

Cloves are not merely a culinary delight; they are a veritable powerhouse of medicinal benefits. These versatile gems harbor a rich array of bioactive compounds, including eugenol, a potent antioxidant that combats free radicals and protects cells from damage. Cloves also boast an impressive array of vitamins and minerals, including vitamin C, vitamin K, and manganese, all of which play crucial roles in maintaining optimal health.

Enhance digestion: Cloves stimulate the production of digestive enzymes, improving nutrient absorption and promoting regularity.

Boost immunity: Cloves' antioxidant and anti-inflammatory properties help strengthen the immune system, protecting against infections and illnesses.

Reduce stress and anxiety: Cloves' calming properties can help soothe the nervous system, promoting relaxation and alleviating stress and anxiety.

7 Cloves Tips Every Woman Should Know

This comprehensive guide unveils the remarkable power of cloves and provides 7 practical tips on how to incorporate these extraordinary buds into your daily life for optimal health and well-being. Discover how cloves can:

1. Enhance your beauty regimen: Harness the power of cloves to

nourish your skin and hair, promoting radiance and vitality.

2. Support respiratory health: Utilize cloves' antibacterial and anti-inflammatory properties to combat respiratory ailments and boost immunity.

3. Promote emotional well-being: Embrace cloves' calming aroma and soothing properties to alleviate stress and anxiety, fostering emotional balance.

4. Enhance your culinary creations: Elevate your culinary

repertoire with cloves, adding a touch of warmth and complexity to your dishes.

5. Craft natural remedies: Discover simple yet effective home remedies using cloves to address common health concerns.

6. Embrace a holistic approach to wellness: Integrate cloves into your daily routine as part of a holistic approach to health and well-being.

7. Empower yourself with knowledge: Become an expert on

the remarkable properties of cloves, empowering yourself to make informed decisions about your health.

Embark on a transformative journey of wellness with 7 Cloves Tips Every Woman Should Know. Unlock the extraordinary power of these aromatic buds and cultivate a life of vibrant health and well-being.

Chapter One

Cloves for Beauty:

<u>A Woman's Guide to Radiant Skin, Hair, and Oral Health</u>

Since time immemorial, women have sought natural remedies to enhance their beauty, scouring the earth for ingredients that could unveil their inner radiance. Among the vast array of natural treasures, cloves, the dried flower buds of the clove tree, have emerged as a hidden gem, offering a wealth of benefits for skin, hair, and oral health.

Cloves for Skin Health: A Natural Elixir for a Radiant Complexion

Cloves, with their potent antibacterial and antiseptic properties, are nature's gift to blemish-free skin. Their rich content of eugenol, a powerful antioxidant, helps combat free radical damage, a major contributor to premature aging. This makes cloves an effective ingredient in anti-aging skincare, reducing the appearance of fine lines and wrinkles, and promoting a youthful glow.

To harness the skin-enhancing properties of cloves, consider incorporating a few drops of clove essential oil into your daily skincare routine. Dilute the oil with a carrier oil, such as jojoba or coconut oil, to prevent skin irritation. Apply the diluted mixture to cleansed skin, focusing on areas of concern, such as blemishes, wrinkles, and dark spots.

Cloves for Hair Health: A Natural Conditioner for Strong and Shiny Locks

Cloves, with their stimulating properties, can revitalize hair from root to tip. Their ability to improve blood circulation to the scalp promotes hair growth and prevents premature hair loss. Additionally, cloves have antifungal properties, helping to combat scalp issues like dandruff and itchy scalp.

To pamper your hair with the goodness of cloves, consider incorporating clove oil into your hair care routine. Add a few drops of clove oil to your regular shampoo or conditioner. You can also prepare a natural hair mask by mixing clove oil with yogurt or honey. Apply the mixture to your hair, massaging it gently into the scalp. After leaving it on for 15 to 20 minutes, give it a good rinse.

Cloves for Oral Health: A Natural Remedy for a Healthy Smile

Cloves, with their antibacterial and analgesic properties, have long been used in traditional medicine to promote oral health. Their ability to combat plaque and gingivitis helps prevent gum disease and bad breath. Additionally, the numbing properties of cloves can provide temporary relief from toothaches.

To maintain oral hygiene and promote a healthy smile, incorporate cloves into your daily routine. Chew on a clove after each meal to freshen your breath and promote oral health. You can also prepare a natural mouthwash by boiling a few cloves in water, allowing the mixture to cool, and then using it to rinse your mouth.

Cloves, with their versatility and efficacy, offer a treasure trove of beauty benefits for women. From promoting radiant skin and healthy hair to maintaining oral health, cloves are a natural ally in a woman's pursuit of inner and outer beauty. Embrace the power of cloves and unveil your natural radiance, one clove at a time.

Chapter 2

Cloves for Health

Cloves, the aromatic flower buds of the clove tree, are a versatile spice with a long history of culinary and medicinal use. Native to Southeast Asia, cloves have been prized for their pungent aroma, warm flavor, and numerous health benefits.

Cloves for Immune System Support

Cloves are a rich source of eugenol, a potent compound with anti-inflammatory and antibacterial properties. Eugenol has been shown to boost the immune system by stimulating the production of white blood cells, which are essential for fighting off infections. Cloves also contain vitamin C, a well-known antioxidant that further enhances immune function.

Cloves for Digestive Health

Cloves have long been used as a digestive aid due to their ability to stimulate digestive juices and promote healthy gut flora. Eugenol has been shown to protect against ulcers and other digestive disorders. Additionally, cloves contain fiber, which helps to regulate bowel movements and prevent constipation.

Cloves for Respiratory Health

Cloves have a warming and expectorant effect, making them an effective remedy for coughs, colds, and bronchitis. Eugenol has been shown to loosen mucus and clear congestion, while other clove compounds have antibacterial and antiviral properties that help to fight off infections.

Cloves for Cardiovascular Health

Cloves may offer protection against heart disease by reducing LDL (bad) cholesterol and increasing HDL (good) cholesterol levels. Eugenol also has antioxidant and anti-inflammatory properties that can help to prevent blood vessel damage.

In addition to these four key health benefits, cloves have also been shown to be beneficial for dental health, pain relief, and blood sugar control.

The following are some pointers for including cloves in your diet:

* Add a few cloves to your morning smoothie or tea
* Ground cloves can be used in baking, sauces, and marinades
* Whole cloves can be chewed on to freshen breath and relieve nausea

* A clove oil diffuser can be used for aromatherapeutic benefits

With their wide range of health benefits and versatility in the kitchen, cloves are a valuable addition to any woman's health and wellness routine.

Chapter 3

Cloves for Emotional Well-being

The fragrant aroma of cloves, a spice commonly used in Indian cuisine, has long been associated with a sense of warmth and comfort. But beyond its culinary appeal, cloves hold a treasure trove of benefits for emotional well-being. This versatile spice has been shown to alleviate stress, reduce anxiety, and enhance mood, making it a valuable tool for women seeking emotional balance and resilience.

Cloves for Stress Relief

Cloves contain eugenol, an active compound with potent anti-inflammatory and analgesic properties. When consumed, eugenol interacts with the body's endocannabinoid system, which plays a crucial role in regulating stress responses. This interaction helps to lower cortisol levels, the body's primary stress hormone, promoting a sense of calm and relaxation.

In addition to their internal action, cloves also offer an external approach to stress relief. The aroma of clove essential oil, when diffused or inhaled, has been shown to activate the parasympathetic nervous system, the branch responsible for relaxation and rest. This calming effect can help ease tension, soothe the mind, and promote better sleep, all of which contribute to stress reduction.

Cloves for Anxiety Relief

The anxiolytic properties of cloves are attributed to their ability to influence the GABAergic system, a neurotransmitter system involved in regulating mood and anxiety. Eugenol, the active compound in cloves, binds to GABA receptors, enhancing the action of GABA and promoting a sense of tranquility.

Cloves also contain caryophyllene, a terpene with anti-anxiety effects. Caryophyllene interacts with the CB2 receptor, part of the endocannabinoid system, and produces a calming effect similar to that of cannabinoids.

Cloves for Mood Enhancement

Cloves possess mood-enhancing qualities that can help combat feelings of sadness, lethargy, and low spirits. Their ability to modulate the GABAergic system and the endocannabinoid system contributes to a more balanced and positive mood. Additionally, cloves contain antioxidants and anti-inflammatory compounds that help reduce oxidative stress and promote overall well-being, which can indirectly influence mood.

Incorporating cloves into your daily routine can significantly enhance your emotional well-being. Here are a few simple ways to reap the benefits of cloves:

* Add a few cloves to your morning cup of tea or herbal infusion.

* Incorporate cloves into your culinary creations, adding a warm and aromatic touch to your meals.

* Diffuse clove essential oil in your home to create a calming and relaxing atmosphere.

Incorporate clove aromatherapy into your massage routine for a deeply soothing and stress-relieving experience.

As you embrace the power of cloves, you'll discover a newfound sense of emotional balance, allowing you to navigate life's challenges with greater resilience and grace. Remember, small steps can lead to significant changes, so start incorporating cloves into your daily life and experience the transformative power of this remarkable spice.

Chapter 4

Cloves in the Kitchen

Cloves, the dried flower buds of the clove tree, have been prized for their culinary and medicinal properties for centuries. Their warm, spicy aroma and pungent flavor have made them a staple in cuisines around the world, from the savory curries of India to the sweet pastries of Europe. In this chapter, we'll explore the versatility of cloves in the kitchen, delving into their use in cooking, baking, and beverage preparation.

Cooking with Cloves:

Cloves' unique flavor profile complements a wide range of savory dishes, adding depth and complexity to meats, stews, soups, and vegetable curries. Their warm, spicy notes harmonize beautifully with other aromatic spices like cinnamon, cardamom, and nutmeg, creating a symphony of flavors that tantalize the taste buds.

Here are some pointers for using cloves in cooking:

1. **Whole Cloves**:Whole cloves are ideal for slow-cooked dishes, where they have time to release their full flavor and aroma. Use them sparingly, as their intensity can be overwhelming.

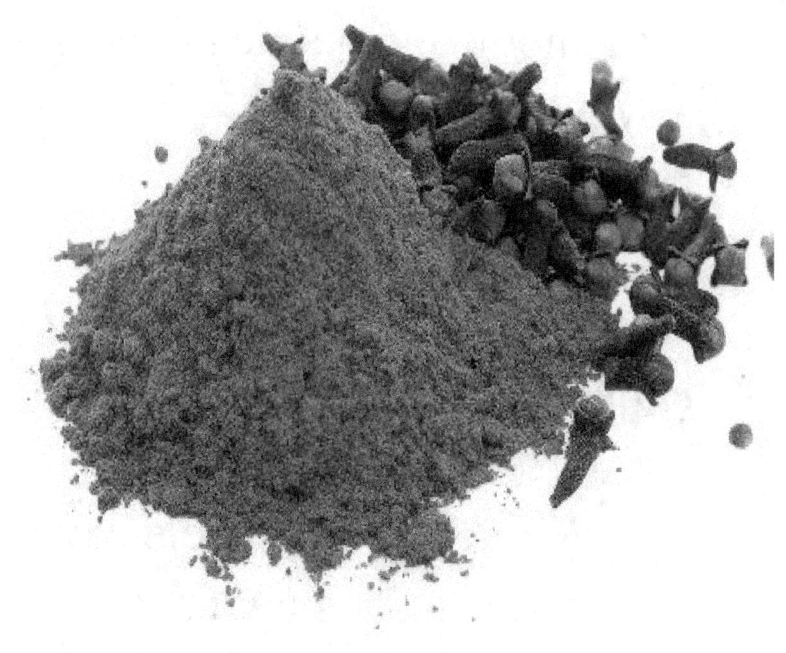

2. **Ground Cloves**: Ground cloves are more versatile, allowing for easier incorporation into recipes. They add a subtle spiciness

and warmth to marinades, rubs, and spice blends.

3. **Clove Infusions**: Cloves can be infused into oils, vinegar, and broths, imparting their distinctive flavor to other ingredients.

Baking with Cloves:

The sweet and spicy essence of cloves makes them a delightful addition to baked goods. They elevate cakes, cookies, pies, and breads with their warm, aromatic touch, adding a touch of sophistication and intrigue.

Here are some tips for baking with cloves:

- **Cloves in Doughs and Batters**: Ground cloves can be incorporated directly into doughs and batters, infusing cakes, cookies, and quick breads with their subtle spiciness.

- **Cloves in Fillings and Frostings**: Cloves can be added to fruit fillings, custards, and frostings, adding depth and complexity to sweet treats.

- **Cloves in Spice Blends**:Cloves are often combined with cinnamon, nutmeg, and ginger in spice blends for pumpkin pie, gingerbread, and other festive treats.

Making Clove-Infused Beverages:

Cloves bring a touch of warmth and spice to beverages, transforming teas, coffees, and mulled wines into aromatic delights. Their invigorating aroma and gentle spiciness make them perfect for sipping on chilly evenings or as a comforting pick-me-up.

Here are some tips for making clove-infused beverages:

*****Clove Tea**:Steep whole cloves in hot water for a fragrant and invigorating tea. Add a touch of honey or lemon for sweetness and balance.

***Clove-Infused Coffee**: Add a few whole cloves to your coffee grounds for a warm, spicy twist. Adjust the amount of cloves to your taste.

***Mulled Wine**: Cloves are a traditional ingredient in mulled wine, adding their distinctive flavor to this festive beverage. Combine cloves with cinnamon, nutmeg, citrus zest, and red wine for a heartwarming treat.

Cloves, with their versatility and unique flavor profile, are a culinary treasure that deserves a place in every kitchen. From savory dishes to sweet treats and comforting beverages, cloves add depth, complexity, and an aromatic touch that elevates any culinary creation. So, embrace the warmth and spice of cloves and let their magic transform your culinary adventures.

Chapter 5

Cloves for Natural Remedies

Cloves, the small, aromatic flower buds of the clove tree, have been used for centuries in traditional medicine for their various health benefits. These versatile spices are not only packed with flavor but also contain a wealth of medicinal properties that can be used to treat a variety of ailments.

Cloves for Toothaches

Toothaches can be excruciating and significantly disrupt your daily life. Cloves, with their potent antibacterial and analgesic properties, can provide natural relief from toothaches. Eugenol, the main constituent of clove oil, acts as a local anesthetic, numbing the affected area and reducing pain.

To use cloves for toothaches, you can:

- Apply a few drops of clove oil directly to the painful

tooth or gum using a cotton swab.

- Prepare a clove paste by grinding a few cloves with a little water or coconut oil. Apply the paste to the affected area and leave it on for 15-20 minutes.

Cloves for Colds and Flu

Cloves have antiviral and antimicrobial properties that can help fight off cold and flu infections. They also act as an expectorant, helping to loosen mucus and clear congestion. To use cloves for colds and flu, you can:

- Inhale the aroma of clove oil by adding a few drops to a diffuser or vaporizer.
- Drink clove tea by steeping a few cloves in hot water. To taste, you can add honey or lemon.
- Gargle with clove water by boiling a few cloves in water and letting it cool down. Gargle with the solution several times a day.

<u>Cloves for Headaches</u>

Headaches can be debilitating and interfere with your daily activities. Cloves, with their anti-inflammatory and analgesic properties, can help ease headache pain. Eugenol, the main component of clove oil, has been shown to be effective in reducing headache symptoms.For headaches, you can use cloves as follows:

- Add a few cloves to a kettle of boiling water and breathe in the steam.

- Apply a few drops of clove oil to your forehead or temples.

- Steep a few cloves in boiling water to make clove tea. To taste, you can add lemon or honey.

Cloves for Stomach Upset

Stomach upset, including indigestion, nausea, and vomiting, can be uncomfortable and disrupt your digestion. Cloves, with their carminative and antispasmodic properties, can help soothe stomach upset and relieve digestive discomfort. To use cloves for stomach upset, you can:

* Drink clove tea by steeping a few cloves in hot water.
*Chew on a few cloves after a meal to aid in digestion.
*Add a few cloves to your cooking for an extra boost of flavor and digestive benefits.

Additional Tips
*Cloves can be used in various forms, including whole cloves, ground cloves, clove oil, and clove tincture.

*Cloves are generally safe for most people when used in moderation. However, some people may experience allergic reactions or skin irritation when using clove oil.

*If you are pregnant or breastfeeding, consult your doctor before using cloves for medicinal purposes.**

By incorporating cloves into your daily routine or using them as a natural remedy for specific ailments, you can reap the benefits of this versatile spice and enhance your overall well-being.

Chapter 6

Cloves in Aromatherapy

Using Cloves Essential Oil for Relaxation

Cloves essential oil has a calming and relaxing effect on the mind and body. It can help to reduce stress, anxiety, and tension. It can also help to improve sleep quality.

To use cloves essential oil for relaxation, you can diffuse it in your home or add it to a bath or massage oil. You can also apply a drop of cloves essential oil to your temples or wrists.

Using Cloves Essential Oil for Pain Relief

Clove essential oil has analgesic properties that can help to relieve pain.It can be used to treat joint discomfort, aches in the muscles, and headaches. Additionally, it can be used to relieve menstruation cramps and toothaches.

To use cloves essential oil for pain relief, you can apply a drop of oil to the affected area. You can also diffuse it in your home or add it to a bath or massage oil.

Using Cloves Essential Oil for Infection Prevention

Clove essential oil has antibacterial and antifungal properties that can help to prevent infections. It can be used to clean wounds, prevent the spread of colds and flu, and treat athlete's foot.

To use cloves essential oil for infection prevention, you can add a few drops of oil to a diffuser or to a spray bottle filled with water. You can also apply a drop of oil to your skin.

Additional Benefits of Cloves Essential Oil

In addition to the benefits listed above, cloves essential oil can also be used to:

* Boost the immune system
* Improve digestion
* Promote healthy skin

* Relieve nausea

Safety Precautions

Cloves essential oil is safe for most people to use. However, it is important to dilute the oil with a carrier oil before applying it to your skin. You should also avoid using cloves essential oil if you are pregnant or breastfeeding.

Chapter 7

Cloves in Everyday Life

<u>Adding Cloves to Your Daily Routine</u>

Cloves are a versatile spice that can be easily incorporated into your daily routine. Here are a few ways to add cloves to your day:

*Add cloves to your morning coffee or tea.Cloves have a warming effect that can help you wake up in the morning. They also have a digestive benefit that can help you get your day started on the right foot.

*Add cloves to your oatmeal or breakfast cereal. Cloves add a sweet and savory flavor to oatmeal and cereal. They can also help to regulate blood sugar levels, which can help you avoid energy crashes throughout the day.
*Add cloves to your soups and stews. Cloves add depth and complexity to soups and stews. They also have antibacterial and

antifungal properties that can help to boost your immune system.

*Add cloves to your desserts. Cloves add a warm and spicy flavor to cakes, cookies, and pies. They can also help to reduce cravings for unhealthy sweets.

*Add cloves to your beauty routine. Cloves can be used to make a natural hair mask or facial scrub. They can also be added to a diffuser to create a relaxing atmosphere.

Making Cloves a Part of Your Self-care Ritual

In addition to their many health benefits, cloves can also be used to promote self-care and relaxation. Here are a few ways to make cloves a part of your self-care ritual:

*Drink a cup of clove tea before bed.Clove tea can help to relax your mind and body and promote a good night's sleep.

* Use clove essential oil in a diffuser.Clove essential oil has a calming and uplifting effect that

can help to reduce stress and anxiety.

*Add cloves to a bath. Cloves can help to relieve muscle aches and pains and promote relaxation.

*Massage clove oil into your skin. Clove oil can help to improve circulation and reduce inflammation.

Sharing the Benefits of Cloves with Others

Cloves are a valuable spice that can benefit everyone. Here are a few ways to share the benefits of cloves with others:

- Cook a meal for your loved ones using cloves. Cloves can add flavor and health benefits to any dish.

- Give a gift of clove essential oil or clove tea. This is a thoughtful and appreciated gift that is sure to be enjoyed.

- Share your knowledge of cloves with others. Talk to your friends and family about the many benefits of cloves.

- Encourage others to use cloves in their daily lives. Cloves are a simple and affordable way to improve your health and well-being.

By incorporating cloves into your daily routine, you can reap the many benefits of this versatile spice. Cloves can help to improve your health, promote relaxation, and boost your overall well-being. So share the benefits of cloves with others and help them to live healthier and happier lives.

Conclusion

Embark on a journey of wellness and embrace the incredible power of cloves, a versatile spice that holds the key to unlocking a healthier, happier life. From its culinary versatility to its remarkable medicinal properties, cloves offer a myriad of benefits that can transform your overall well-being.

Indulge in the rich aroma and flavor of cloves, adding a touch of culinary magic to your favorite dishes. Whether you're simmering a hearty stew, baking fragrant cookies, or brewing a soothing cup of tea, cloves infuse your creations with a unique warmth and depth of flavor.

Venture beyond the realm of cuisine and discover the remarkable healing properties of cloves. Harness its potent antibacterial and anti-inflammatory effects to soothe a sore throat, ease digestive discomfort, or alleviate menstrual cramps. The natural compounds found in cloves also possess antioxidant and immune-boosting qualities, supporting your body's defenses against illness.

As you embrace the power of cloves, you'll not only enhance your culinary creations but also cultivate a healthier, more vibrant life. Let the aroma of cloves fill your kitchen, signaling the start of a journey toward a more wholesome and balanced existence.